This is a booklet is formulated to be used as reference only. Fruits provide certain health benefits that have been researched and documented. When added together they form a synergy that surpasses the individual components. In other words the sum is greater than the whole of their parts. It is a smart company that can put their resources together and add these special super fruits to their already patented formula of a naturally occurring matrix of collagen.

Did you know that all diseases come from inflammation?

What if you could reduce your future health care costs, naturally?

This booklet is the author's composite, and not the efforts of anyone else. The author found it necessary to share the benefits of specific Super Fruits and show they can benefit others.

This booklet was produced with the intention for the individual to read and use for personal preference.

Super Fruits that at the very least help to;

- support a healthy immune system,
- protect DNA,
- Reduce oxidative stress

Super Fruits are packed with Phytonutrients that provide a wide-range of biological activities and amazing Anti-inflammatory benefits.

While you are looking through this book, circle the fruits that stand out for you. If you would like to know about a specific product that the author is aware of that has all these fruits, please contact; Chris Marcelle at info@ahealthandwellnessco.com or 321-258-5916

A	B	C
acai	astragalus	acerola
apple	kiwi	mangosteen
blueberry	apple	acai
cranberry	pear	amla
goji	pineapple	apple
jujube	pomegranate	cranberry
mangosteen	rhiodiola	goji
maqui	strawberry	grape
noni	tart cherry	jabuticaba
pomegranate		maqui
red grapes		pear
strawberry		pomegranate
		schisandra

Super Fruits found in Blend A

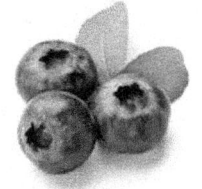

Blueberry (Bilberry) Blueberries for many years, blueberries have been used for medicinal purposes. The combination of the fiber and the pectin content has proven to lower blood cholesterol. The research has concluded that the most effective medicinal use for Bilberry/Blueberry extract appears to be improving micro-circulation. Improving micro-circulation in turn aids the capillaries that serve the eyes, and mucous membranes of the digestive and pulmonary systems. Improved capillaries increase circulation to the connective tissue which may help people that suffer from arthritis, water retention in the legs, varicose veins, bruising and hemorrhoids. Blueberries also contain measurable quantities of ellagic acid, which has been proven to prevent chemically induced cancer in laboratory studies.

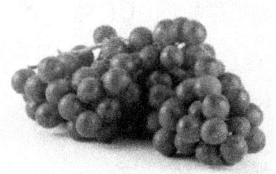

Grape Resveratrol is found in Grapes. Research shows that Resveratrol plays an important part in anti-aging and anti-cancer activity. Resveratrol is a potent anti-oxidant and has the capability to inhibit platelet aggregation. These two characteristics may help prevent free radical damage throughout the body and provide protective support to the cardiovascular system. There continues to be research on the benefits of resveratrol. Research suggests that resveratrol strongly inhibits blood pressure, heart rate, and renal sympathetic nerve activity. The Zhejiang University in China investigated the effect of resveratrol on the central regulation of blood pressure, heart rate, and renal sympathetic nerve activity in animals. This study has tremendous implications for anti-aging therapies. Grapes create one of the main detoxifying foods. There is a wide range of benefits found in Grapes, including vision improvement, supportive for circulatory problems, hypertension, arteriosclerosis, and rheumatic illnesses such as gout and arthritis.

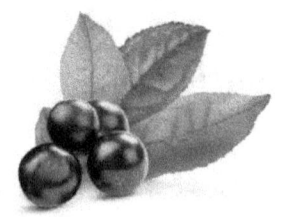

Maqui berries are very rich in anthocyanins, which are purple pigments with very high antioxidant activity. Specifically, maqui berries contain high levels of anthocyanins called delphinidins, which is also found in violas, delphiniums, and Concord grapes. But in maqui berry, these compounds are found in unusually high amounts. The delphinidins demonstrate potent anti-inflammatory activity, so they help to reduce the risk of a variety of degenerative diseases that involve inflammation. These pigments also inhibit the growth of colon cancer cells. Inflammation is part of virtually every degenerative disease, from cardiovascular disease to diabetes to arthritis. Any illness that ends with "itis" is an inflammatory disease. The anthocyanins exhibit powerful anti-inflammatory activity, and do it as well as drugs for the same purposes, without negative effects.

The antioxidant compounds in maqui berry help prevent the oxidation of cholesterol in the blood. Oxidation of cholesterol is a factor in the development of cardiovascular disease, including heart attack, stroke and hardening of the arteries. Regular daily intake of maqui berries or the berry juice is a wise decision for better cardiovascular health. Remarkably, intake of maqui berries or their juice causes a significant increase of insulin in the body. In fact, maqui appears to do this better than any other known plant. Consuming maqui berries or their juice with or after meals can help to overpower blood glucose. Therefore, maqui may prove to be a beneficial aid in weight control. Maqui also exhibits antibacterial activity, which suggests that it may support in preventing illness due to foodborne germs.

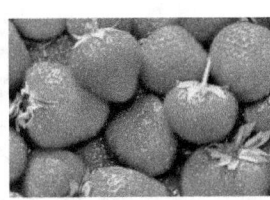

Strawberry

Strawberries are an excellent foundation of Vitamin C, manganese, dietary fiber, iodine, potassium, folate, vitamin B5, Vitamin B6, and Vitamin K, riboflavin, omega-3 fatty acids, magnesium and copper. Ellagic acid found in Strawberries knowingly reduces cancer cells. Ellagic acid prevents the destruction of P53 gene by cancer cells and can also bind with cancer causing molecules making them inactive. Like many other berries, Strawberries contain high amounts of anti-oxidants; in particular anthocyanins and ellagitannins. These compounds help to neutralize the destructive effects of free radicals. Strawberries inhibit the inflammatory process; and can reduce the rate of mutation in cells. A serving of Strawberries will provide you with 200mg of potassium, which may help regulate the electrolytes in your body, lowering your risk of heart attack and stroke. Strawberries have been used for sunburn, discolored teeth, digestion, and gout. As far back as the 13th century, the Strawberry was used as an aphrodisiac. Strawberries were served at medieval state events; they symbolized prosperity, peace, and perfection.

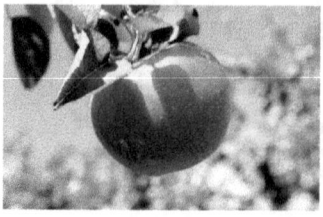

Apples are naturally fat-free, cholesterol-free and sodium-free. An apple a day keeps the doctor away! Whoever came up with that saying wasn't kidding. Apples are packed with a storehouse of vitamins and nutrients, which can enhance your immune system and help ward off diseases. Apples contain plenty of anti-oxidants like flavonoids and polyphenols, which are useful in the body for guarding it against various toxic substances and disease-causing germs. It is an excellent source of B-complex vitamins for mental and cardiovascular functioning. Apples offer better energy production; immune enhancement; anti-cholesterol properties; anti-inflammatory; an excellent source of fiber; offers protection from free radicals; and pectin in Apples help in controlling blood sugar levels; and Apples are considered useful for gall bladder and kidney stone problems.

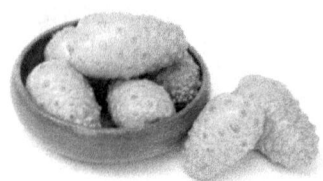

Noni has habitually been used for colds, flu, diabetes, anxiety, and hypertension, as well as an antidepressant and anxiolytic. All plant parts are used for a variety of illnesses in Samoan culture, and noni is one of the most frequently used Hawaiian plant medicines. Claims that have often been unsubstantiated in clinical trials include: the use of bark for the treatment of bacterial infections, cough, diarrhea in infants, and stomach ailments; the flowers for sore or irritated eyes, sties, conjunctivitis, ocular inflammation, and coughs; the fruit for asthma, wounds, broken bones, mouth and throat infections, tuberculosis, worms, diarrhea, fever, vomiting, eye ailments, arthritis, depression, seizures, bacterial and fungal infections, viruses, and as a tonic; the fresh fruit juice for cancer; the dried leaves used externally for infections, burns, children's chest colds, and inflammation, and internally for boils, pleurisy, inflamed gums, and arthritic pain; the fresh leaves used externally for burns and internally for fevers, hemorrhage, bacterial infections, and inflammation; and the roots for oral ulcerations, fevers, and cancerous swellings.

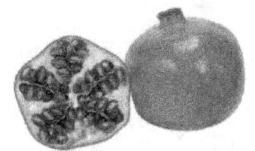 **Pomegranates** astringent properties have been used to treat various ailments, such as cuts, sore throats, tapeworms, dysentery, and gum disease. Pomegranate juice is marketed in the U.S. as a major source of antioxidant nutrients that protect against heart disease and other ailments. Recent research has focused on its potential use as a treatment for cardiovascular disease, diabetes, and various forms of cancer. The potent anti-oxidant properties of the fruit have been accredited to its high content of soluble polyphenols. When tested in vitro on normal and colon-cancer cell lines, the juice was found to have superior anti-oxidant, anti-proliferative, and pro-apoptotic effects. Other studies show excellent outcome on bone and cartilage; and excellent effect in the cosmetic arena, showing stimulation of a type of procollagen synthesis and inhibition of dermal degeneration processes. For centuries pomegranates have been regarded as a treasure among fruits. Babylonians and ancient Egyptians held them in the highest regard as a wonder fruit. Pomegranates are often referred to as the jewel of winter and people who five years ago had never even heard of the fruit are now excited about its potential health benefits.

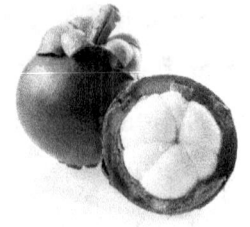

Mangosteen The medicinal properties of

the Mangosteen fruit are derived mainly from its outer rind or peel, not from the inner part of the fruit. The rind, called the 'pericarp' is where powerful anti-oxidants are highly concentrated. You might notice tiny particles of the pericarp when you drink Jusuru. This is the medicinal part of the Mangosteen. These unique anti-oxidants, known as Xanthones, have properties which help to heal cells damaged by free radicals, slow aging, and ward off degenerative diseases and physical and mentaldeterioration. According to research reported in professional journals, these amazing xanthones have a remarkably beneficial effect on cardiovascular health. The key to the mangosteen is that it's one of the only sources of xanthones. Xanthones are among the most powerful antioxidants to be found in nature. Xanthones are biologically active plant phenols found in a few select tropical plants.Current research on xanthones suggests they are beneficial in helping with many conditions including: allergies, infections (microbial,fungus, viral), cholesterol levels, skin disorders, gastro-intestinal disorders, and fatigue. They are also naturally antibiotic, antiviral, and anti-inflammatory.

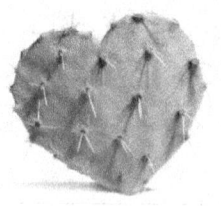

Nopal The ability for the prickly pear cactus

(nopal) to lower blood sugar has been well documented by many studies. In traditional Mexican medicine, nopal is used for treating type-2 Diabetes.

Mexican researchers found that people with non-insulin-dependent diabetes given broiled nopal stems experienced a large drop in blood sugar levels.

It has been shown that daily consumption of 250mg of this plant will lower total cholesterol and LDL cholesterol levels, according to a recent study. HDL cholesterol and triglyceride levels were not affected.

In India, the cactus has been used to treat whooping cough and asthma. Prickly pear fruit and other elements of the cactus are edible as a jelly or jam, as a fruit or as a cooked dish.

The cactus is naturally found in Arizona, Mexico and other parts of the American Southwest; it is commercially grown in California and also has been exported to Europe and India.

In the Sonoran Desert, growing a new prickly pear is easy: the cactus grows in a linked "pad" setup, and each pad can be cut off, replanted and in most cases will take root, making a new cactus.

For many diabetics or prediabetics, nopal is a complete replacement for prescription blood sugar drugs. It regulates blood sugar with no negative side effects and no liver damage (which is one of the primary side effects of blood sugar prescriptions). Safety note: Do not halt prescription drug use except under the direct supervision of a naturopathic physician.

Nopal is a key ingredient is many highly effective (and safe) blood sugar regulating nutritional supplements (see resources, below). Conventional medicine, including drug companies and the FDA, do not want the public to learn about nopal because it would cost Big Pharma hundreds of millions of dollars in annual profits from diabetes drug sales. The public is intentionally kept ignorant about natural treatments for diabetes as a way to maximize corporate profits.

Most doctors have never heard of nopal, or its ability for blood sugar balancing effects, because the use of medicinal herbs is simply not taught in medical school. Virtually all M.D.s are nutritionally illiterate when it comes to herbs and food supplements.

Native Americans, who are suffering under an epidemic of diabetes, desperately need to be re-taught the medicinal uses of desert plants. If nopal were widely harvested and used to help regulate blood sugar in Native Americans, the diabetes rate would fall sharply. But conventional medicine, dominated primarily by rich white men, chooses to deliberately deny honest information about nutritional supplements to Native Americans. In doing so, Native Americans have been isolated from their land and their medicinal wisdom.

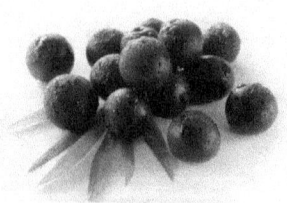

Acai Berry Rich in carbohydrates, vitamins, minerals, proteins, and fat, making it nature's perfect food. Acai berry contains the following essential ingredients: Vitamin B1 (Thiamin), Vitamin B2 (Riboflavin), Vitamin B3 (Niacin), Vitamin C, Vitamin. E ,(Tocopherol), iron, potassium, phosphorus, and calcium. People have been using Acai berry to get that age-defying beauty, energy, improved vision, stronger heart, and better mental clarity, just to mention a few of the benefits. In addition, regular use of the berries can help you lose weight and get rid of the toxins. People have also been using this fruit since the time it was discovered to be a natural cholesterol controller. It reduces bad cholesterol in our blood and increases the good cholesterol. The açaí is a high-energy berry that grows wild in the Amazon Rainforest and has been the staple source of vitamins and nutrients for the native Amazonian people for centuries. Açaí tastes like a vibrant blend of berries and chocolate and is packed full of antioxidants, amino acids, and essential fatty acids. Research on the açaí berry has focused on its antioxidant activity. The açaí berry contains anthocyanin. The word anthocyanin comes from two Greek words meaning plant and blue. Anthocyanins are responsible for the red, purple, and blue hues in many fruits, vegetables, and flowers. Foods that are richest in anthocyanins -- such as blueberries, red grapes, red wine, and açaí -- are very strongly colored, ranging from deep purple to black. In addition to anthocyanins, açaí contains flavonoids. Anthocyanins and flavonoids are powerful antioxidants that help defend the body against life's stressors. They also play a role in the body's cell protection system. Eating a diet rich in antioxidants may interfere with the aging process by neutralizing free radicals. By lessening the destructive power of free radicals, antioxidants help keep your body healthy.

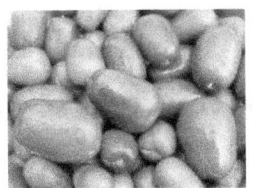 **Jujube** The medicinal properties of Jujube fruit have been known and used for more than 4,000 years. The fruit has very high vitamin C content. According to the National Center for Biotechnology, juice from the Jujube fruit has been shown to have cytotoxic activity on different tumor lines. These benefits have been attributed to, among other things, the Jujube's high content of bioactive compounds. Studies conducted over a 20 year period have shown bioactive compounds to play an important role in the prevention of chronic diseases. Jujube fruit is also an anti-oxidant with rejuvenating properties. It has the ability to help clear up the skin. The fruits contain saponin, alkaloids and triterpenoids. These three compounds are all beneficial in purifying the blood, and as an aid to digestion. Although most Americans haven't heard of it yet, the jujube (Ziziphus jujuba) is legendary in China. It's a tree that's been cultivated in the Shandong province for over 4,000 years. It produces a delicious fruit that contains so much nutritional value that it's reputed that priests lived on nothing but jujube fruit for

years at a time. It's this astonishing nutrient-rich essence that has caused the jujube fruit to come to be known as "the fruit of immortality". For thousands of years, the jujube fruit and its juice have been prized for their amazing health and medicinal values. In the very first textbook of Chinese herbalism, jujube was given a prominent role. Written by the founder of Chinese herbal medicine, this ancient text praised and recommended jujube for its ability to cleanse the blood of toxins, cleanse the kidneys, liver, heart, and other vital organs, and build stamina and energy. In addition to its rich nutritional value, the jujube is also said to have great healing properties for those suffering from illness or less than ideal health. Prized for thousands of years in China, and long considered almost a complete food in itself, and a powerful healing agent.

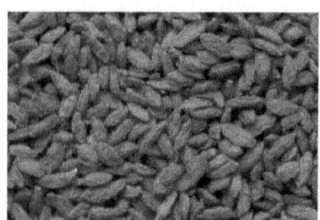

Goji berries (Lycium barbarum) are the most nutritionally dense fruit on Earth. They are a member of the nightshade family (Solonaceae), which contains many other common vegetables such as potato, tomato, eggplant, and pepper, as well as some poisonous plants like belladonna and deadly nightshade. Native to the Himalayan Mountains of Tibet and Mongolia, the goji berry is now grown in many other countries as well. Although they have only been introduced in Western countries in recent years, gojis have been used for thousands of years in Tibet and China, both as a culinary ingredient and medicinally. Unique among fruits because they contain all essential amino acids, goji berries also have the highest concentration of protein of any fruit. They are also loaded with vitamin C, contain more carotenoids than any other food, have twenty-one trace minerals, and are high in fiber. Boasting 15 times the amount of iron found in spinach, as well as calcium, zinc, selenium and many other important trace minerals, there is no doubt that the humble goji berry is a nutritional powerhouse.

This amazing little super fruit also contains natural anti-inflammatory, anti-bacterial and anti-fungal compounds. Their powerful antioxidant properties and polysaccharides help to boost the immune system. It's no wonder then, that in traditional Chinese medicine they are renowned for increasing strength and longevity.

In traditional Chinese medicine, the goji is said to act on the Kidney and Liver meridians to help with lower back pain, dizziness and eyesight. They are most often consumed raw, made into a tea or extract, or as an ingredient in soups.

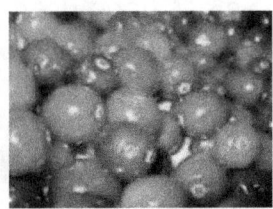

Cranberry Cranberries medicinal properties
have been recognized for centuries Native Americans used raw Cranberries as a wound dressing; for digestive problems; blood disorders, and scurvy (Vitamin C deficiency). Cranberries are an excellent source of Vitamin C. Cranberries are high in anti-oxidants and contain a potent vasodilator. Recent studies have shown it can reduce the ability of E.coli to adhere to the lining of the bladder and urethra, reducing the potential for urinary tract infections. Further studies indicated that Cranberries also prevent another microorganism known as heliobacter pylori from adhering to cell walls. H.pylori is a bacterium that can cause stomach ulcers. Studies also suggest that Cranberries may help prevent bacteria from adhering to gums and around the teeth.

Super Fruits found in B

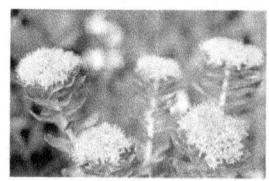

Rhodiola rosea has been used in traditional medicine as a means to stimulate the nervous system, decrease depression and fatigue for centuries in Eastern Europe and Asia. It is also used to help prevent high altitude sickness. Rhodiola rosea is believed to offer many different kinds of health benefits, it is known as "golden root". Rhodiola rosea is a plant in the Crassulaceae family; it has separate female and male plants. Rhodiola rosea is classified as an adaptogen; adaptogen is an agent increases in power of resistance against multiple stressors and helps the body to reassume homeostasis. Rhodiola rosea has been used for centuries to cope with the cold Siberian climate and stressful life. Rhodiola rosea promotes the release of certain neurotransmitters responsible for feelings of well-being, as well as regulating hormone production in response to stress including oxidative damage by free radicals. Rhodiola rosea also appears to increase the permeability of the blood-brain barrier to neurotransmitter precursors, aiding and even increasing their beneficial effects. Rhodiola rosea has been studied extensively in the last few years and this herb may have multiple health benefits. Liver Rhodiola rosea may offer benefits to liver; it has been used to protect the liver in traditional medicine for years.

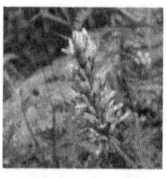

Astragalus is a unique immunity boosting herb native to China and Mongolia. In Chinese medicine astragalus health benefits have been put to treat common colds and flu due to high content of active compounds like polysaccharides, saponins and flavonoids. To get a full spectrum of benefits, astragalus extract is manufactured using a whole plant including its roots.

Let's take a look at top 10 astragalus health benefits and which health conditions it can help improve.

1. Digestive astragalus health benefits are demonstrated in lowering excessive acidity of the stomach, increasing body's metabolic rates and promoting faster waste elimination pattern. This is incredibly beneficial for people suffering from stomach ulcers and acid indigestion.

2. Astragalus tea should be regularly consumed during common flu and cold seasons starting in early fall and through the winter. Astragalus health benefits help increase white blood cell count, stimulate growth of antibodies and elevate body's resistance to bacteria and viruses.

3. Astragalus health benefits go beyond common ailments and can even enhance traditional chemotherapy treatments in cancer patients. Astragalus extract and tea taken throughout cancer treatment will help lessen the side effects from such treatments and boost patient's immune system.

4. Astragalus root health benefits work to protect you from high blood pressure, arrhythmia and generally improve your cardiac function.

5. Astragalus extract helps you keep your cholesterol counts in check. Astragalus tea works by preventing fatty plaque deposits in arteries to allow blood to flow freely. In addition, astragalus prevents fats from being absorbed from the intestines and facilitates their accelerated evacuation from the body.

6. Astragalus was shown effective to treat various forms of anemia and improving hemopoietic (blood making) function.

7. Patients who have been diagnosed with HIV and AIDS could draw incredible benefits from using astragalus based medicine. Active compounds found in this herb could support patients' immune systems and even be used in place of common HIV drugs. However, more research is still needed in this field.

8. Astragalus health benefits also encompass herpes simplex virus that is a culprit behind recurring oral herpes outbreaks. People affected by oral herpes notice fewer outbreaks while taking astragalus extract.

9. Astragalus is very often used in combination with other herbal supplements to treat chronic nephritis and various stages of renal failure. Patients treated with a combo of astragalus and rehmannia root showed improvement as to lower levels of protein and blood in urine.

10. Astragalus is a very important ingredient for managing diabetes in Chinese medicine. Not only this herb helps lowering blood sugar, it also prevents pathological changes in the retina, blood vessels, enhances liver and kidney function.

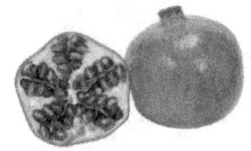

Pomegranates astringent properties have been used to treat various ailments, such as cuts, sore throats, tapeworms, dysentery, and gum disease. Pomegranate juice is marketed in the U.S. as a major source of antioxidant nutrients that protect against heart disease and other ailments. Recent research has focused on its potential use as a treatment for cardiovascular disease, diabetes, and various forms of cancer. The potent anti-oxidant properties of the fruit have been attributed to its high content of soluble polyphenols. When tested in vitro on normal and colon-cancer cell lines, the juice was found to have superior anti-oxidant, anti-proliferative, and pro-apoptotic effects. Other studies show excellent effect on bone and cartilage; and excellent effect in the cosmetic arena, showing stimulation of a type of procollagen synthesis and inhibition of dermal degeneration processes. For centuries pomegranates have been regarded as a treasure among fruits. Babylonians and ancient Egyptians held them in the highest regard as a wonder fruit. Pomegranates are often referred to as the jewel of winter and people who five years ago had never even heard of the fruit are now excited about its potential health benefits.

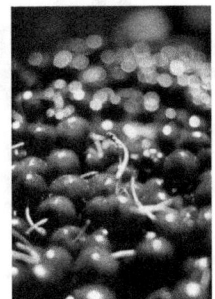 **Tart cherries** are loaded with important nutrients, but you'd have to eat an entire bag of them to obtain all of the benefits you can get by sipping the juice. The fruit also contains many antioxidants and anti-inflammatory agents, and its juice aids in cancer prevention and heart health and as an anti-inflammatory, which can help alleviate a variety of ailments like asthma symptoms and pain. In short, tart cherry juice offers protection against a host of conditions. Tart Cherries Contain Important Phytonutrients Called Anthocyanins. Tart cherries, like all red fruits and vegetables, are rich in anthocyanins, a class of antioxidant phytochemical (a disease-fighting agent found in plant-based foods). Other fruits and vegetables in this class include raspberries, strawberries, beets, cranberries, apples, red onions, kidney beans and red beans. Phytochemicals give brightly colored fruits and vegetables their colorful hues. Anthocyanins, in particular, encourage

healthy circulation, ensure proper nerve function and offer cancer fighting properties.

Antioxidant Benefits of Tart Cherry Juice

Consumption of tart cherry juice provides older adults greater protection against the development of heart disease, cancer and age-related cognitive decline, according to a research study published in August 2009 by the Journal of Nutrition. In the study,

"Tart Cherry Juice Decreases Oxidative Stress in Healthy Older Men and Women," researchers Tinna Traustadóttir, Sean S. Davies, Anthoney A. Stock and others investigated whether the consumption of foods high in anthocyanins is associated with improved health, in particular if the consumption of tart cherry juice (high in anthocyanins) improves the ability of older adults to resist oxidative damage.

Oxidative damage may lead to an increased rate of death and disease in the elderly in response to infections, and diseases such as atherosclerosis, cancer, diabetes and Alzheimer's disease.

"The roles of anthocyanin pigments as medicinal agents have been well-accepted dogma in folk medicine throughout the world, and, in fact, these pigments are linked to an amazingly broad-based range of health benefits," says Mary Ann Lila in an article titled "Anthocyanins and Human Health: An In Vitro Investigative Approach" published in a 2004 issue of the Journal of Biomedicine and Biotechnology.

"For example, anthocyanins have historically been used in remedies for liver dysfunction and hypertension; and bilberry (Vaccinium) anthocyanins have an anecdotal history of use for vision disorders, microbial infections, diarrhea, and diverse other health disorders," wrote Lila, who currently serves as director of North Carolina State University's Plants for Human Health Institute.

Clinical research trials later supported the anecdotal and epidemiological evidence of the use of anthocyanins for therapeutic purposes, the researcher went on to say, noting "some reports suggest that anthocyanin activity is potentiated when delivered in mixtures" -- that is, a juice blend may provide even greater results.

BENEFIT #1: Tart Cherry Juice Provides Extra Cancer Protection

Carcinogens, harmful substances in air, water and foods, may damage the body's cells, triggering changes that may lead to cancer. Tart cherry juice offers more than anthocyanins; it is loaded with three disease-fighting chemicals that may be beneficial for halting cell transformation (that often leads to cancer). These powerful chemicals are perillyl alcohol, limonene and ellagic acid. Citrus peel offers limonene and berries offer ellagic acid, but only cherries offer all three chemicals. They are particularly protective against cancers of the breast, lung, liver and skin.

"Anthocyanins have demonstrated marked ability to reduce cancer cell proliferation and to inhibit tumor formation," Lila said. "Fruit extracts with significant anthocyanin concentrations proved to be effective against various stages of carcinogenesis."

Though the perillyl alcohol does show promise, according to the American Institute for Cancer Research, researchers still have much to learn about dose, methods of delivery, as well as how to identify who might benefit most.

BENEFIT #2: Quercetin in Tart Cherry Juice Helps Fight Heart Disease

Tart cherry juice contains one of the most powerful antioxidants that exists, quercetin. Among other functions, quercetin prevents oxidative damage caused by free radicals from damaging low-density lipoprotein (LDL or "bad" cholesterol), according to a study published in European Review for Medical and Pharmacological Science in 2013. When LDL cholesterol is oxidized, it is more likely to adhere to artery walls, forming plaque which contributes to heart attack and stroke.

Numerous studies cite the effectiveness of quercetin in reducing blood pressure, but also call for more research on the correlation between consumption of the flavonoid and such health benefits.

"In one study, intake of high levels of quercetin was associated with reduced incidence of type 2 diabetes," note authors of a 2013 study published in International Journal of Preventive Medicine.

"In vitro studies showed different effects of quercetin as anti-inflammatory, antioxidant, anti-clotting, and vasodilatory properties. But, human and animal studies did not have consistent results, which may result from different physiology of species and also different levels of oxidative stress and inflammatory status," according to Maryam Zahedi, Reza Ghiasvand, Awat Feizi, Gholamreza Asgari and Leila Darvish in the article "Does Quercetin Improve Cardiovascular Risk factors and Inflammatory Biomarkers in Women with Type 2 Diabetes: A Double-blind Randomized Controlled Clinical Trial."

BENEFIT #3: Tart Cherry Juice Protects Against Muscle Damage

One study tested the efficacy of a tart cherry juice blend in preventing the symptoms of exercise-induced muscle damage in 14 male college students. The dosage was 12 ounces of a cherry juice blend or a placebo taken twice daily for eight days with a series of elbow flexion contractions performed on the fourth day of supplementation.

Pain and strength loss were significantly lower in the cherry juice trial versus placebo, according to "Efficacy of a Tart Cherry Juice Blend in Preventing the Symptoms of Muscle Damage" published in a December 2006 issue of the British Journal of Sports Medicine by researchers D.A. Connolly, M.P. McHugh and O.I. Padilla-Zakour.

"Most notably, strength loss averaged over the four days after eccentric exercise was 22 percent with the placebo but only 4 percent with the cherry juice. These results have important practical applications for athletes, as performance after damaging exercise bouts is primarily affected by strength loss and pain. In addition to being an efficacious treatment for minimizing symptoms of exercise induced muscle damage, consumption of cherry juice is much more convenient than many of the treatments that have been presented in the literature," the researchers say.

BENEFIT #4: Tart Cherry Juice Aids in Sports Recovery

In related findings, marathon runners who consumed 8 ounces of tart cherry juice twice a day for five days prior to a marathon, on the day of the marathon and for 48 hours after the run experienced less muscle damage, soreness, inflammation and protein breakdown than runners who consumed a placebo, according to research published in the December 2010 issue of the Scandinavian Journal of Medicine and Science in Sports.

Runners who consumed 11 to 12 ounces of tart cherry juice twice daily for seven days prior to a long-distance relay and during the 24 hours of the race reported significantly less pain following the run than those who consumed a placebo, according to another study, published in a 2010 issue of the Journal of the International Society of Sports Nutrition.

BENEFIT #5: Arthritis Sufferers May Benefit From Tart Cherry Juice's Anti-Inflammatory Properties

Drinking a glass of tart cherry juice in the morning and the evening may be a better and a safer way to treat insomnia and add nearly 90 minutes of sleep to your night, according to researchers at Louisiana State University.

Tart cherries are a natural source of melatonin, a hormone that helps regulate the sleep-wake cycle, say Frank L. Greenway, MD, director of the outpatient research clinic at the LSU Pennington Biomedical Research Center, and Jack Losso and John Finley, professors in the School of Nutrition and Food Sciences at the university's Agricultural Center in their study, "Tart Cherry Juice Increases Sleep Time in Older Adults with Insomnia" presented at Experimental Biology 2014.

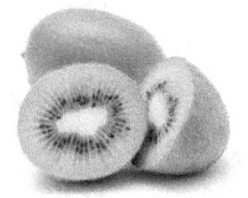 **Kiwifruit** consuming fruits and vegetables of all kinds has long been associated with a reduced risk of heart disease, diabetes, cancer and other conditions. Many studies have shown that increased consumption of plant foods like kiwis decreases the risk of obesity and overall mortality. A Kiwifruit is rich in vitamin C

Beautiful Skin: Collagen, the skins support system, is reliant on vitamin C as an essential nutrient that works in our bodies as an antioxidant to help prevent damage caused by the sun, pollution and smoke, smooth wrinkles and improve overall skin texture. Better Sleep: According to a study on the effects of kiwifruit consumption on sleep quality in adults with sleep problems, it was found that kiwi consumption may improve sleep onset, duration, and efficiency in adults with self-reported sleep disturbances.

Heart Health: The fiber and potassium in kiwis support heart health. An increase in potassium intake along with a decrease in sodium intake is the most important dietary change that a person can make to reduce their risk of cardiovascular disease, according to Mark Houston, MD, MS, an associate clinical professor of medicine at Vanderbilt Medical School and director of the Hypertension Institute at St Thomas Hospital in Tennessee. In one study, those who consumed 4069 mg of potassium per day had a 49% lower risk of death from ischemic heart disease compared with those who consumed less potassium (about 1000 mg per day).High potassium intakes are also associated with a reduced risk of stroke, protection against loss of muscle mass, preservation of bone mineral density and reduction in the formation of kidney stones.

Lowering Blood Pressure: Kiwis have high potassium content, as a result, kiwis can help negate the effects of sodium in the body. It is possible that a low potassium intake is just as big of a risk factor in developing high blood pressure as a high sodium intake. According to the National Health and Nutrition Examination Survey, fewer than 2% of US adults meet the daily 4700 mg recommendation for potassium.

Also of note, a high potassium intake is associated with a 20% decreased risk of dying from all causes. Constipation Prevention: Numerous studies have reported that the kiwi may have a mild laxative effect and could be used as a dietary supplement especially for elderly individuals experiencing constipation. Regular consumption of kiwifruit was shown to promote bulkier, softer and more frequent stool production

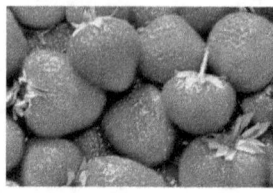 **Strawberry** are an excellent foundation of Vitamin C, manganese, dietary fiber, iodine, potassium, folate, vitamin B5, Vitamin B6, and Vitamin K, riboflavin, omega-3 fatty acids, magnesium and copper. Ellagic acid found in Strawberries knowingly reduces cancer cells. Ellagic acid prevents the destruction of P53 gene by cancer cells and can also bind with cancer causing molecules making them inactive. Like many other berries, Strawberries contain high amounts of anti-oxidants; in particular anthocyanins and ellagitannins. These compounds help to neutralize the destructive effects of free radicals. Strawberries inhibit the inflammatory process; and can reduce the rate of mutation in cells. A serving of Strawberries will provide you with 200mg of potassium, which may help regulate the electrolytes in your body, lowering your risk of heart attack and stroke. Strawberries have been used for sunburn, discolored teeth, digestion, and gout. As far back as the 13th century, the Strawberry was used as an aphrodisiac. Strawberries were served at medieval state events; they symbolized prosperity, peace, and perfection.

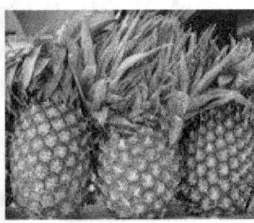

Pineapple or "ananas" has an interesting history to narrate. Originally indigenous to local Paraguayans in South America, it spread from its native land by the local Indians up through the South and Central Americas and to the West Indies. Later, it was brought to Spain when Columbus discovered Americas' in 1493. In the 15th and 16th centuries, it spread to rest of the world by the European sailors (just like tomatoes) who carried it along with them to protect themselves from scurvy, a disease caused by the deficiency of vitamin C. Scientifically, it is known as "Ananas comosus" and belongs to the family of Bromeliaceae, in the genus; Ananas. Pineapple is a tropical, perennial, drought-tolerant plant. it grows up to 5-8 ft in height and spreads around about 3-4 feet radius cover. It is essentially a short, stout stem with a rosette of waxy long, needle-tipped leaves.

Health benefits of Pineapple fruit

Fresh pineapple is low in calories. Nonetheless, it is a storehouse for several unique health promoting compounds, minerals and vitamins that are essential for optimum health.100 g fruit provides just about 50 calories equivalent to that of apples. Its flesh contains no saturated fats or cholesterol; however, it is rich source of soluble and insoluble dietary fiber like pectin.

Pineapple fruit contains a proteolytic enzyme bromelain that digests food by breaking down protein. Bromelain also has anti-inflammatory, anti-clotting and anti-cancer properties. Studies have shown that consumption of pineapple regularly helps fight against arthritis, indigestion and worm infestation.

Fresh pineapple is an excellent source of antioxidant vitamin; vitamin C. 100 g fruit contains 47.8 or 80% of this vitamin. Vitamin C is required for the collagen synthesis in the body. Collagen is the main structural protein in the body required for maintaining the integrity of blood vessels, skin, organs, and bones. Regular consumption of foods rich in vitamin C helps the body protect from scurvy; develop resistance against infectious agents (boosts immunity) and scavenge harmful, pro-inflammatory free radicals from the body.

It also contains small amount Vitamin A (provides 58 IU per 100 g) and beta-carotene levels. These compounds are known to have antioxidant properties. Vitamin A is also required maintaining healthy mucusa, skin and is essential for vision. Studies suggest that consumption of natural fruits rich in flavonoids helps the human body to protect from lung and oral cavity cancers.

In addition, ananas fruit is rich in B-complex group of vitamins like folates, thiamin, pyridoxine, riboflavin and minerals like copper, manganese and potassium. Potassium is an important component of cell and body fluids, helps controlling heart rate and blood pressure. Copper is a helpful cofactor for red blood cell synthesis. Manganese is a co-factor for the enzyme superoxide dismutase, which is a very powerful free radical scavenger.

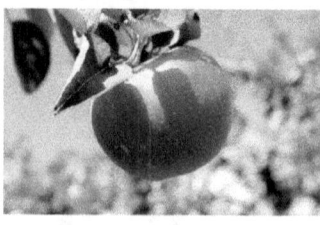 **Apples** are naturally fat-free, cholesterol-free and sodium-free. An apple a day keeps the doctor away! Whoever came up with that saying wasn't kidding. Apples are packed with a

storehouse of vitamins and nutrients, which can enhance your immune system and help ward off diseases. Apples contain plenty of anti-oxidants like flavonoids and polyphenols, which are useful in the body for guarding it against various toxic substances and disease-causing germs. It is an excellent source of B-complex vitamins for mental and cardiovascular functioning. Apples offer better energy production; immune enhancement; anti-cholesterol properties; anti-inflammatory; an excellent source of fiber; offers protection from free radicals; and pectin in Apples help in controlling blood sugar levels; and Apples are considered useful for gall bladder and kidney stone problems

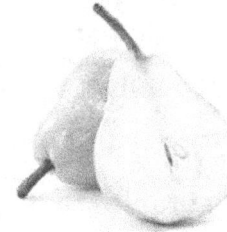

Pears are such a valuable source of food that people would sometimes include the word Perry in place names to indicate that pears were growing there. Here are eight health benefits of pears that may make you want to eat them more often.

Immune System Booster
A strong immune system is essential in fighting off disease and illness. Pears help to boost the immune system because they contain antioxidants such as vitamin C and copper which fight off free radicals and disease in the body.

Osteoporosis Prevention
Preventing and treating osteoporosis is a major concern for many people. Many doctors are now recommending that people who are concerned with protecting the health of their bones maintain a balanced ph and high calcium intake from dietary sources. Fruits and vegetables help to maintain a healthy pH level and pears are a good

source of boron, which researchers believe may help the body to retain calcium.

Increased Energy Levels

when you eat a pear, your body absorbs glucose, which is converted into energy. Eating a pear can be a great pick-me-up if you feel sluggish in the afternoon.

Digestive Health

Pears contain a lot of fiber, which is essential for a healthy digestive system. Fiber helps to keep food moving efficiently through the colon. One medium sized pear contains about 20-25% of the daily recommended intake of fiber. A good percentage of the fiber in pears is insoluble, which may help to reduce the occurrence of colon polyps.

Cancer Prevention

One way to prevent cancer is by eating fresh fruits and vegetables that are high in antioxidants. Pears contain vitamin C, a powerful antioxidant which is an important part of your body's cancer fighting arsenal. The fiber content in pears is very effective at promoting colon health which will reduce your chances of developing colon cancer.

Healthy Pregnancy

In order to avoid birth defects, it is important for pregnant women to consume enough folic acid. Pears contain 10-20 mcg (about 5% of the RDA) of the natural form of folic acid, folate, and they should be included in a healthy prenatal diet.

Less Allergenic

Pears are considered by some people to be a hypoallergenic food, which is why they are often recommended to people who suffer from food allergies and weaning babies. However, they are not completely hypoallergenic, as some people do have allergic reactions to pears, particularly those people who are allergic to Alder or Birch pollen.

Good for Weaning

many doctors recommend pears for babies when they are weaning and being introduced to baby food. This is because pears are a low acid fruit that are unlikely to cause digestion problems in little bellies and because pear allergy is relatively rare.

Super Fruits found in C

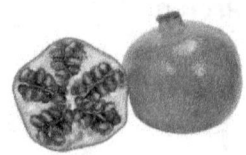

Pomegranates astringent properties have been used to treat various ailments, such as cuts, sore throats, tapeworms, dysentery, and gum disease. Pomegranate juice is marketed in the U.S. as a major source of antioxidant nutrients that protect against heart disease and other ailments. Recent research has focused on its potential use as a treatment for cardiovascular disease, diabetes, and various forms of cancer. The potent anti-oxidant properties of the fruit have been accredited to its high content of soluble polyphenols. When tested in vitro on normal and colon-cancer cell lines, the juice was found to have superior anti-oxidant, anti-proliferative, and pro-apoptotic effects. Other studies show excellent outcome on bone and cartilage; and excellent effect in the cosmetic arena, showing stimulation of a type of procollagen synthesis and inhibition of dermal degeneration processes. For centuries pomegranates have been regarded as a treasure among fruits. Babylonians and ancient Egyptians held them in the highest regard as a wonder fruit. Pomegranates are often referred to as the jewel of winter and people who five years ago had never even heard of the fruit are now excited about its potential health benefits.

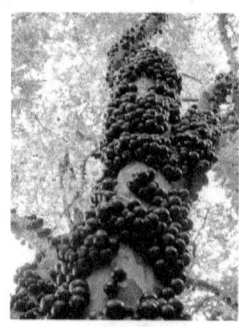

Jaboticaba is a fruit that is low in fat, low in calories and low in carbohydrates. It is a rich source of vitamin C and also contains other vitamins like vitamin E, thiamine, niacin, riboflavin and folic acid. Minerals like calcium, potassium, magnesium, iron, phosphorus, copper, manganese and zinc are also present in this fruit. In addition to vitamins and minerals, Jaboticaba is also a good source of several amino acids, fatty acids and many powerful antioxidants that have anti-cancer and anti-inflammatory properties.

Jaboticaba is a good addition to a weight loss diet since it is low in fat and calories. Besides, the skin is a rich source of dietary fiber that controls your appetite and prevents you from overeating by keeping you fuller for a longer period of time. Jabuticaba Fruit has been found to have strong astringent properties. It helps in opening up the bronchial air passages and hence is a good remedy for asthma the astringent effects also makes it effective in treating diarrhoea and inflammation of the tonsillitis. The high levels of calcium, potassium and magnesium in this fruit is beneficial for your bones and teeth. These minerals help in strengthening your bones and in preventing conditions like osteoporosis. They are eaten raw, although one shouldn't eat the skins as they are very astringent because they have high tannin content, which could be harmful if eaten in large quantities for a prolonged period of time. They are eaten raw or used to make jams and marmalades, although they have to have added pectin to set. Wine can also be made from the fruit which can be sweet or slightly acid and astringent, depending on the variety

Jaboticaba is a fruit that is low in fat, low in calories and low in carbohydrates. It is a rich source of vitamin C and also contains other vitamins like vitamin E, thiamin, niacin, riboflavin and folic acid. Minerals like calcium, potassium, magnesium, iron, phosphorus, copper, manganese and zinc are also present in this fruit. In addition to vitamins and minerals, Jaboticaba is also a good source of several amino acids, fatty acids and many powerful antioxidants that have anti-cancer and anti-inflammatory properties.

Studies reveal that Jabotica peel is a high source of dietary fiber and phenolic compounds (anthocyanins) that have potent antioxidant properties. Jabuticaba along with its Myrtaceae family fruits have high content of ellagitannins. Jabuticaba peel has one of the highest content of ellagic acid. Anthocyanins content increases with ripening of the fruit.

Health benefits of Jaboticaba

Being a rich source several important nutrients, the health benefits of Jaboticaba are numerous and promising too. Some of the benefits are listed below:

Antioxidant properties of Jaboticaba

Jaboticaba has high content of phenolic compounds and antioxidants. The oxidation stress caused by the free radicals to the cells of your body is mainly responsible for ageing and also many health conditions like cancer. Antioxidants help in getting rid of these free radicals and in preventing cell damage. Research is active in the area of antioxidant properties of jaoticaba.

Jaboticaba and skin benefits

Being one of the powerful antioxidants it prevent early aging and also in preventing the occurrence of ageing signs like dark spots, wrinkles and fine lines. This exotic fruit has important nutrients, especially in its peel that has been found to be very beneficial for your skin. Studies have found that Jaboticaba helps in rejuvenating and hydrating your skin. It also encourages the production of collagen that helps in increasing the elasticity and suppleness of skin. The pulp of this fruit contains vitamin B3 (Niacinamide) which supports the functioning of enzymes that promote cell growth. It also has detoxifying and anti-microbial properties and hence is used in the treatment of acne. Jaboticaba is used in preparation of tropical skin care formulations. Mix jaboticaba pulp, oatmeal and honey to make jaboticaba face scrub at home.

Jaboticaba for healthy hair. The nutrients in Jaboticaba promote healthy and lustrous growth of hair and are also helpful in preventing hair loss. Various formulations with Jaboticaba extract for hair are also available in market.

Jaboticaba and weight loss. Jaboticaba is a good addition to a weight loss diet since it is low in fat and calories. Besides, the skin is a rich source of dietary fiber that controls your appetite and prevents you from overeating by keeping you fuller for a longer period of time.

Jaboticaba has anti-cancer properties. Jabuticaba is very popular for its powerful antioxidant effects due to the presence of phenolic compounds like anthocyanins and many others. Anthocyanins, which act as potent antioxidants also possess anti-inflammatory, with anti-cancer properties. These antioxidants help in fighting off the free radicals that are responsible for causing cell damage and DNA mutations.

Jaboticaba has strong astringent properties. Jabuticaba Fruit has been found to have strong astringent properties. It helps in opening up the bronchial air passages and hence is a good remedy for asthma The astringent effects also makes it effective in treating diarrhea and inflammation of the tonsilitis.

Jaboticaba and digestive health. The high fiber content in Jaboticaba helps in making your bowel movements regular and in preventing constipation. The nutrients in this fruit aid in digestion and also in cleansing and detoxifying your intestine.

Jaboticaba may help in reducing cardiovascular diseases. It has been found that diets rich in anthocyanin or polyphenols can lower your risks of cardiovascular diseases by regulating lipid metabolism. A study conducted in obese rats confirmed that such diets help in reducing the total serum cholesterol and triglyceride levels and also in increasing the good cholesterol (HDL) levels. Jaboticaba peel is a rich source of dietary fiber that is capable of lowering the levels of LDL and total cholesterol.

Jaboticaba and diabetes. According to studies conducted on mice, the peel of Jaboticaba is effective in reducing blood glucose levels and hence its regular consumption may be helpful in preventing type 2 diabetes. Since it a low calorie food with plenty of dietary fiber, it is a healthy addition to the diet of people with diabetes. Animal studies have also found out anti-obesity properties of jaboticaba peel.

Jabuticaba for stronger bones and teeth. The high levels of calcium, potassium and magnesium in this fruit is beneficial for your bones and teeth. These minerals help in strengthening your bones and in preventing conditions like osteoporosis.

Jaboticaba relieves arthritis. Because of its powerful anti-inflammatory properties, Jaboticaba is useful in easing arthritis and other inflammation related disorders.

Jaboticaba is good for pregnant women. In olden times, Jaboticaba was given to pregnant women because of the high amounts of iron in it.

This fruit is also a good source of folic acid that plays a major role in the growth and development of the baby.

Jaboticaba is a good source of depside. Depsides are polyphenolic compounds that exhibit antioxidant, antibiotic, anti-HIV and anti-proliferative properties. A depside known as jaboticabin has been found to be present in Jaboticaba, which is considered to play a key role in promoting health benefits.

Regular consumption of Jaboticaba ensures that your body gets the essential vitamins and minerals needed for maintaining normal and healthy bodily functions.

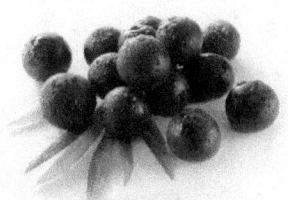 **Acai Berry** Rich in carbohydrates, vitamins, minerals, proteins, and fat, making it nature's perfect food. Acai berry contains the following essential ingredients: Vitamin B1 (Thiamin), Vitamin B2 (Riboflavin), Vitamin B3 (Niacin), Vitamin C, Vitamin. E , (Tocopherol), iron, potassium, phosphorus, and calcium. People have been using Acai berry to get that age-defying beauty, energy, improved vision, stronger heart, and better mental clarity, just to mention a few of the benefits. In addition, regular use of the berries can help you lose

weight and get rid of the toxins. People have also been using this fruit since the time it was discovered to be a natural cholesterol controller. It reduces bad cholesterol in our blood and increases the good cholesterol. The açaí is a high-energy berry that grows wild in the Amazon Rainforest and has been the staple source of vitamins and nutrients for the native Amazonian people for centuries. Açaí tastes like a vibrant blend of berries and chocolate and is packed full of antioxidants, amino acids, and essential fatty acids.

Research on the açaí berry has focused on its antioxidant activity. The açaí berry contains anthocyanin. The word anthocyanin comes from two Greek words meaning plant and blue. Anthocyanins are responsible for the red, purple, and blue hues in many fruits, vegetables, and flowers. Foods that are richest in anthocyanins -- such as blueberries, red grapes, red wine, and açaí -- are very strongly colored, ranging from deep purple to black. In addition to anthocyanins, açaí contains flavonoids. Anthocyanins and flavonoids are powerful antioxidants that help defend the body against life's stressors. They also play a role in the body's cell protection system. Eating a diet rich in antioxidants may interfere with the aging process by neutralizing free radicals. By lessening the destructive power of free radicals, antioxidants help keep your body healthy.

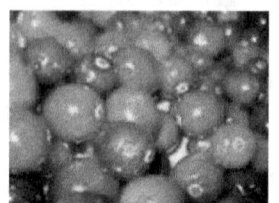 **Cranberry** medicinal properties have been recognized for centuries Native Americans used raw Cranberries as a wound dressing; for digestive problems; blood disorders, and scurvy (Vitamin C deficiency). Cranberries are an excellent source of Vitamin Cranberries are high in anti-oxidants and contain a potent vasodilator. Recent studies have shown it can reduce the ability of E.coli to adhere to the lining of the bladder and urethra, reducing the potential for urinary tract infections. Further studies indicated that Cranberries also prevent another microorganism known as helicobacter pylori from adhering to cell walls. H.pylori is a bacterium that can cause stomach ulcers. Studies

also suggest that Cranberries may help prevent bacteria from adhering to gums and around the teeth.

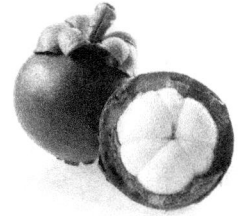

Mangosteen The medicinal properties of the Mangosteen fruit are derived mainly from its outer rind or peel, not from the inner part of the fruit. The rind, called the 'pericarp' is where powerful anti-oxidants are highly concentrated. You might notice tiny particles of the pericarp when you drink Jusuru. This is the medicinal part of the Mangosteen. These unique anti-oxidants, known as Xanthones, have properties which help to heal cells damaged by free radicals, slow aging, and ward off degenerative diseases and physical and mentaldeterioration. According to research reported in professional journals, these amazing xanthones have a remarkably beneficial effect on cardiovascular health. The key to the mangosteen is that it's one of the only sources of xanthones. Xanthones are among the most powerful antioxidants to be found in nature. Xanthones are biologically active plant phenols found in a few select tropical plants. Current research on xanthones suggests they are beneficial in helping with many conditions including: allergies, infections (microbial,fungus, viral), cholesterol levels, skin disorders, gastro-intestinal disorders, and fatigue. They are also naturally antibiotic, antiviral, and anti-inflammatory

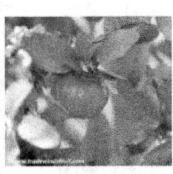

Acerola and is one of the richest sources of vitamin C. Acerola is used as a source of food and juice. Because of its high concentration of vitamin C, it also is sold as a natural

health supplement. Acerola provides other useful vitamins and minerals. Acerola contains from 1 to 4.5 percent vitamin C (1,000 to 4,500 mg/100 g) in the edible portion of the fruit. This far exceeds the content of vitamin C in peeled oranges (about 0.05 or 50 mg/100 g) Antioxidant Vitamin C is known to strengthen the immune system and build collagen cells. It also supports the respiratory system. Vitamin C is known to be an effective antioxidant. The antioxidative qualities of acerola make it an ideal ingredient in skin care products to fight cellular aging. In another report, acerola extract was shown to enhance the antioxidant activity of soy and alfalfa extracts, acting synergistically. This may be beneficial in coronary artery disease.

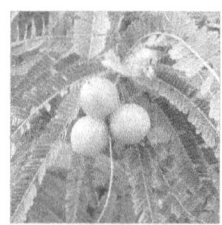 **Amla**, better known as Indian Gooseberry, is widely used in the Ayurvedic medicine system of India. Amla is extremely rich in vitamin C, having thirty percent more than oranges. It's packed with many vitamins, minerals, tannins and other helpful nutrients.This herb is a very powerful antioxidant, preventing damage from free radicals that cause cell oxidation. Antioxidants are important for anti-aging and preventing diseases such as cancer, diabetes and heart disease. Amla also works well for inflammation. It is a good anti-inflammatory for joints especially. This potent herb is also used to reduce fevers, strengthen the heart, control blood sugar, treat urinary tract infections and improve eyesight. Due to the fact that it contains a high amount of fiber, it's also beneficial for problems such as constipation. Amla helps to promote regular bowel movements. Besides the already mentioned health benefits of Amla, it is also great for reducing stress. It helps the

body to calm down and relax. Many people use it to treat insomnia for this reason. Amla is said to improve fertility, strengthen the lungs and boost the immune system, making it more capable in fighting off diseases. It is also often used for sunburns and sun stroke. This herb is considered an exfoliating and astringent agent. Regular use will make the skin look younger. It is helpful to reduce skin sagging, as it tightens the skin. It is often used to prevent hair loss and to keep hair from turning grey. It can make hair more lustrous and healthy looking.

Amla is good for strong bones, teeth and nails, as it helps the body absorb calcium.

Amla Uses:

- As a powerful antioxidant
- Make the skin tighter and younger
- For anti-aging
- Treat cancer
- Treat diabetes
- Treat heart disease
- Treat urinary tract infections
- Good source of fiber
- Treat infections
- Treat eye problems
- Reduce stress
- Relieve constipation
- As an anti-inflammatory
- Helpful for joints
- Treat insomnia
- Improve fertility
- Strengthen the lungs
- Boost the immune system
- Treat sunburn and Sun stroke
- Make skin look younger
- As an exfoliating and astringent agent
- Reduce skin sagging and tighten the skin

- Prevent hair loss

- Prevent grey hair

- Promote strong bones, teeth and nails

- Regulate blood sugar

- Inhibiting the HIV virus

- Prevent respiratory ailments such as common cold, bronchitis

- Treat gastritis

- Improve eyesight

- Remove toxins

- Lower cholesterol

- Maintain liver health

- Increase red blood cell count

- Treat hemorrhage

- Treat diarrhea and dysentery

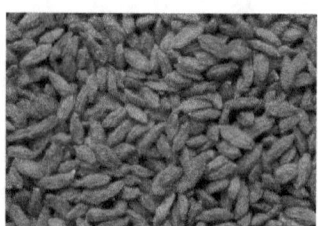

Goji berries (Lycium barbarum) are the most nutritionally dense fruit on Earth. They are a member of the nightshade family (Solonaceae), which contains many other common vegetables such as potato, tomato, eggplant, and pepper, as well as some poisonous plants like belladonna and deadly nightshade. Native to the Himalayan Mountains of Tibet and Mongolia, the goji berry is now grown in many other countries as well. Although they have only been introduced in Western countries in recent years, gojis have been used for thousands of years in Tibet and China, both as a culinary ingredient and medicinally.

Unique among fruits because they contain all essential amino acids, goji berries also have the highest concentration of protein of any fruit. They are also loaded with vitamin C, contain more carotenoids than any other food, have twenty-one trace minerals, and are high in fiber. Boasting 15 times the amount of iron found in spinach, as well as calcium, zinc, selenium and many other important trace minerals, there is no doubt that the humble goji berry is a nutritional powerhouse.

This amazing little super fruit also contains natural anti-inflammatory, anti-bacterial and anti-fungal compounds. Their powerful antioxidant properties and polysaccharides help to boost the immune system. It's no wonder then, that in traditional Chinese medicine they are renowned for increasing strength and longevity.

In traditional Chinese medicine, the goji is said to act on the Kidney and Liver meridians to help with lower back pain, dizziness and eyesight. They are most often consumed raw, made into a tea or extract, or as an ingredient in soups.

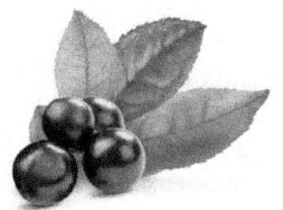

Maqui berries are very rich in

anthocyanins, which are purple pigments with very high antioxidant activity. Specifically, maqui berries contain high levels of anthocyanins called delphinidins, which is also found in violas, delphiniums and Concord grapes. But in maqui berry, these compounds are found in unusually high amounts. The delphinidins demonstrate potent anti-inflammatory activity, so they help to reduce the risk of a variety of degenerative diseases that involve inflammation. These pigments also inhibit the growth of colon cancer cells. Inflammation is part of virtually every degenerative disease, from cardiovascular disease to diabetes to arthritis. Any illness that ends with "itis" is an inflammatory disease. The anthocyanins exhibit powerful anti-inflammatory activity, and do it as well as drugs for the same purposes, without negative effects.

The antioxidant compounds in maqui berry help to prevent the oxidation of cholesterol in the blood. Oxidation of cholesterol is a factor in the development of cardiovascular disease, including heart attack, stroke and hardening of the arteries. Regular daily intake of maqui berries or the berry juice is a smart investment in better cardiovascular health. Interestingly, intake of maqui berries or their juice causes a significant increase of insulin in the body. In fact, maqui appears to do this better than any other known plant. What does this mean? Consuming maqui berries or their juice with or after meals can help to suppress blood glucose, thereby evening out energy and preventing the formation of new fat cells. As a result, maqui may prove to be a beneficial aid in weight control.Maqui also demonstrates antibacterial activity, which suggests that it may aid in preventing illness due to foodborne germs. The Mapuche native people have been eating maqui berries and drinking their juice for centuries. And other non-native people in Chile have done the same for a very long time as well. Even in an environment in which the maret is literally flooded with so-called super fruits, maqui stands head and shoulders above most of them in terms of benefits.

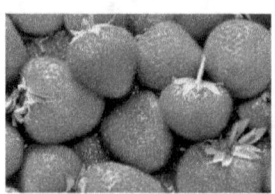 **Strawberry** are an excellent source of Vitamin C, manganese, dietary fiber, iodine, potassium, folate, vitamin B5, Vitamin B6, and Vitamin K,

riboflavin, omega-3 fatty acids, magnesium and copper. Ellagic acid found in Strawberries significantly reduces cancer cells. Ellagic acid prevents the destruction of P53 gene by cancer cells and can also bind with cancer causing molecules making them inactive. Like many other berries, Strawberries contain high amounts of anti-oxidants; in particular anthocyanins and ellagitannins. These compounds help to neutralize the destructive effects of free radicals. Strawberries inhibit the inflammatory process; reduce the rate of mutation in cells. A serving of Strawberries will provide you with 200mg of potassium, which may help regulate the electrolytes in your body, lowering your risk of heart attack and stroke. Strawberries have been used for sunburn, discolored teeth, digestion, and gout. As far back as the 13th century, the Strawberry was used as an aphrodisiac. Strawberries were served at medieval state events; they symbolized prosperity, peace, and perfection. American Indians allegedly invented Strawberry shortcake, mashing berries in meal to make bread the colonists enjoyed--but they must have used wild strawberries since strawberries have been cultivated in America only since 1835.

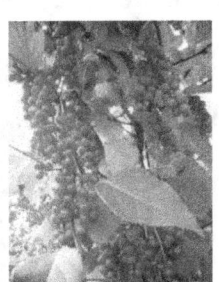

Schizandra (sometimes spelled Schisandra) berries
are a powerful adaptogen. This means that they will help you adapt to your environment allowing you to better handle stress, whether mental or physical. An adaptogen is used as an overall wellness tonic. It is beneficial to the whole body. Like any adaptogen, Schizandra exerts a normalizing effect on the entire body. It will take you from any extreme back to a balanced state. In China, it is said to be the most protective of

all herbs and plants. Schizandra can have a very beneficial impact on your health. It can increase capacity for physical and mental exercise and protect you from environmental stress.

This herb can increase your energy by stimulating the central nervous system without making you nervous like caffeine would. But since it's an adaptogen, it can also calm the nervous system when facing stress.

Many people take this herb to increase energy. It is especially popular with athletes as it boosts nitric oxide levels in the body. It fights fatigue as well, making it even more beneficial. Schizandra increases energy at the cellular level.

The Health Sciences Institute states that schizandra berry can raise the body's enzyme, glutathione. This enzyme detoxifies the body in a way that improves mental clarity. It is widely taken by students in China for this reason.

Probably its best known property is as a protector of the liver, due to the lignans it contains. It helps maintain its proper functioning and regeneration and is also used to prevent liver damage. Schizandra uses its fat soluble compounds found in the core of its seed to protect the liver from toxins.

Schizandra is often used in the treatment of hepatitis C. Besides its liver protecting properties, it is also beneficial to the kidneys as it helps balances the fluid in the body.

This amazing herb also contains antioxidants, such as gomisin A and Wuweizisu C, to protect your cells from free radicals and prevent oxidation. This is why it's often used in longevity formulas in Chinese medicine.

Schizandra is very popular among woman for its ability to make the skin soft, smooth and beautiful. It has been taken for many hundreds of years in China for this purpose. It is believed to work by balancing the fluids of the skin.

This herb is popular with people who suffer from mental disorders such as anxiety, depression and mood swings. Though it's unknown how it works for these symptoms, Schizandra has been used for these ailments for many hundreds of years with much success.

Though not enough research has been done in this area, there is some preliminary evidence that Schizandra my inhibit cancer cell growth for some types of cancers, such as leukemia. Much more research needs to be done before this will be considered a truly effective treatment.

For men, this herb may be beneficial for impotence and erectile dysfunction since it has the ability to dilate the blood vessels, helping men achieve erection.

As far as heart health goes, this herb's blood vessel dilating properties are also good for lowering blood pressure, improving circulation and improving heart function in general.

Schizandra is beneficial to the respiratory system too. It rids the body of lung mucus by acting as expectorant. It is also used to treat coughs.

Schizandra Uses

- As a powerful adaptogen
- Increase strength and stamina
- Increase energy
- For clarity of mind
- Fight fatigue
- Treat asthma
- Treat influenza
- Treat premenstrual syndrome
- Help digestion and treat indigestion
- Treat liver disease
- Enhance the working of the immune system
- As a powerful antioxidant
- Treat respiratory ailments
- Improve the functioning of the respiratory system
- As an aphrodisiac
- For anti-aging and longevity
- Treat sore throats, colds and coughs
- Protect the liver and lungs
- Treat insomnia and night sweats
- Treat mental and physical exhaustion
- Relieve stress
- Treat depression
- Increase circulation
- Treat high blood pressure
- Recuperation following surgery
- For it's anti-bacterial and anti-viral properties
- treat chronic fatigue syndrome
- Protect and enhance vision and hearing
- Treat insomnia
- Lower high cholesterol
- Treat asthma

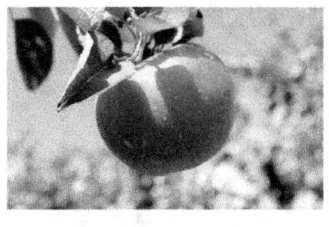

Apples are naturally fat-free, cholesterol-free and sodium-free. An apple a day keeps the doctor away! Whoever came up with that saying wasn't kidding. Apples are packed with a storehouse of vitamins and nutrients, which can enhance your immune system and help ward off diseases. Apples contain plenty of anti-oxidants like flavonoids and polyphenols, which are useful in the body for guarding it against various toxic substances and disease-causing germs. It is an excellent source of B-complex vitamins for mental and cardiovascular functioning. Apples offer better energy production; immune enhancement; anti-cholesterol properties; anti-inflammatory; an excellent source of fiber; offers protection from free radicals; and pectin in Apples help in controlling blood sugar levels; and Apples are considered useful for gall bladder and kidney stone

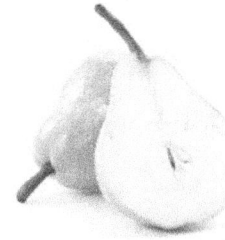

Pears are such a valuable source of food that people would sometimes include the word Perry in place names to indicate that pears were growing there. Here are eight health benefits of pears that may make you want to eat them more often.

Immune System Booster
A strong immune system is essential in fighting off disease and illness. Pears help to boost the immune system because they contain antioxidants such as vitamin C and copper which fight off free radicals and disease in the body.

Osteoporosis Prevention

Preventing and treating osteoporosis is a major concern for many people. Many doctors are now recommending that people who are concerned with protecting the health of their bones maintain a balanced ph and high calcium intake from dietary sources. Fruits and vegetables help to maintain a healthy pH level and pears are a good source of boron, which researchers believe may help the body to retain calcium.

Increased Energy Levels

When you eat a pear, your body absorbs glucose, which is converted into energy. Eating a pear can be a great pick-me-up if you feel sluggish in the afternoon.

Digestive Health

Pears contain a lot of fiber, which is essential for a healthy digestive system. Fiber helps to keep food moving efficiently through the colon. One medium sized pear contains about 20-25% of the daily recommended intake of fiber. A good percentage of the fiber in pears is insoluble, which may help to reduce the occurrence of colon polyps.

Cancer Prevention

One way to prevent cancer is by eating fresh fruits and vegetables that are high in antioxidants. Pears contain vitamin C, a powerful antioxidant which is an important part of your body's cancer fighting arsenal. The fiber content in pears is very effective at promoting colon health which will reduce your chances of developing colon cancer.

Healthy Pregnancy

In order to avoid birth defects, it is important for pregnant women to consume enough folic acid. Pears contain 10-20 mcg (about 5% of the

RDA) of the natural form of folic acid, folate, and they should be included in a healthy prenatal diet.

Less Allergenic
Pears are considered by some people to be a hypoallergenic food, which is why they are often recommended to people who suffer from food allergies and weaning babies. However, they are not completely hypoallergenic, as some people do have allergic reactions to pears, particularly those people who are allergic to Alder or Birch pollen.

Good for Weaning
Many doctors recommend pears for babies when they are weaning and being introduced to baby food. This is because pears are a low acid fruit that are unlikely to cause digestion problems in little bellies and because pear allergy is relatively rare.

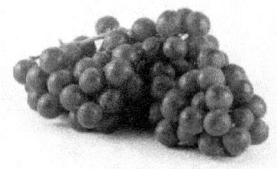

Grape Research shows that Resveratrol, found in Grapes has great potential in anti-aging and anti-cancer activity. Resveratrol has potent anti-oxidant activity and also has the ability to inhibit platelet aggregation. These actions may help prevent free radical damage throughout the body and provide protective support to the cardiovascular system. The research continues to find many more interesting benefits from this compound. Researchers at Zhejiang University in China investigated the effect of resveratrol on the central regulation of blood pressure, heart rate, and renal sympathetic nerve activity in animals. Their results suggest that resveratrol powerfully inhibits blood pressure, heart rate, and renal sympathetic nerve activity. This study has tremendous implications for anti-aging therapies. Grapes constitute one of the main detoxifying foods. Grapes have a wide range of beneficial properties including vision enhancement, helpful for circulatory problems, hypertension, arteriosclerosis, rheumatic illnesses such as gout and arthritis. It is the red grape that we use in our proprietary JUSURU Life Blend that has such powerful health benefits.

Fruits listed in the Individual Products

References

http://altmedicine.about.com/od/completeazindex/a/schisandra.htm

http://altmedicine.about.com/od/completeazindex/a/tart_cherry.htm

http://thehealthyeatingsite.com/the-health-benefits-of-goji-berries/

http://www.doctoroz.com/article/astragalus-root-right-you

http://www.drugs.com/npc/acerola.html

http://www.drugs.com/npp/jujube.html

http://www.foxnews.com/health/2011/01/26/marvelous-maqui-berry.html

http://www.herbcyclopedia.com/item/myrciaria-cauliflora-and-the-benefits
-of-anthocyanins-2

http://www.herbslist.net/amla.html

http://www.herbwisdom.com/herb-rhodiola.html

http://www.naturalhomecures.net/mangosteen/?bingmangosteenkw

http://www.naturalnews.com/021626.html

http://www.nutrition-and-you.com/pineapple.html

http://www.webmd.com/vitamins-supplements/ingredientmono-758-NONI.aspx?
activeIngredientId=758&activeIngredientName=NONI

http://www.webmd.com/vitamins-supplements/ingredientmono-958-CRANBERRY.aspx? activeIngredientId=958&activeIngredientName=CRANBERRY

http://www.whfoods.com/genpage.php?tname=foodspice&dbid=15

http://www.whfoods.com/genpage.php?tname=foodspice&dbid=28

http://www.whfoods.com/genpage.php?tname=foodspice&dbid=32

http://www.whfoods.com/genpage.php?tname=foodspice&dbid=40

http://www.whfoods.com/genpage.php?tname=foodspice&dbid=41

http://www.whfoods.com/genpage.php?tname=foodspice&dbid=8

https://www.organicfacts.net/health-benefits/fruit/health-benefits-of-acai-berries.html

For more information call or email today!

Chris Marcelle, MBA
321-258-5916
www.chrismarcelle.com
www.ahealthandwellnessco.com
info@ahealthandwellnessco.com